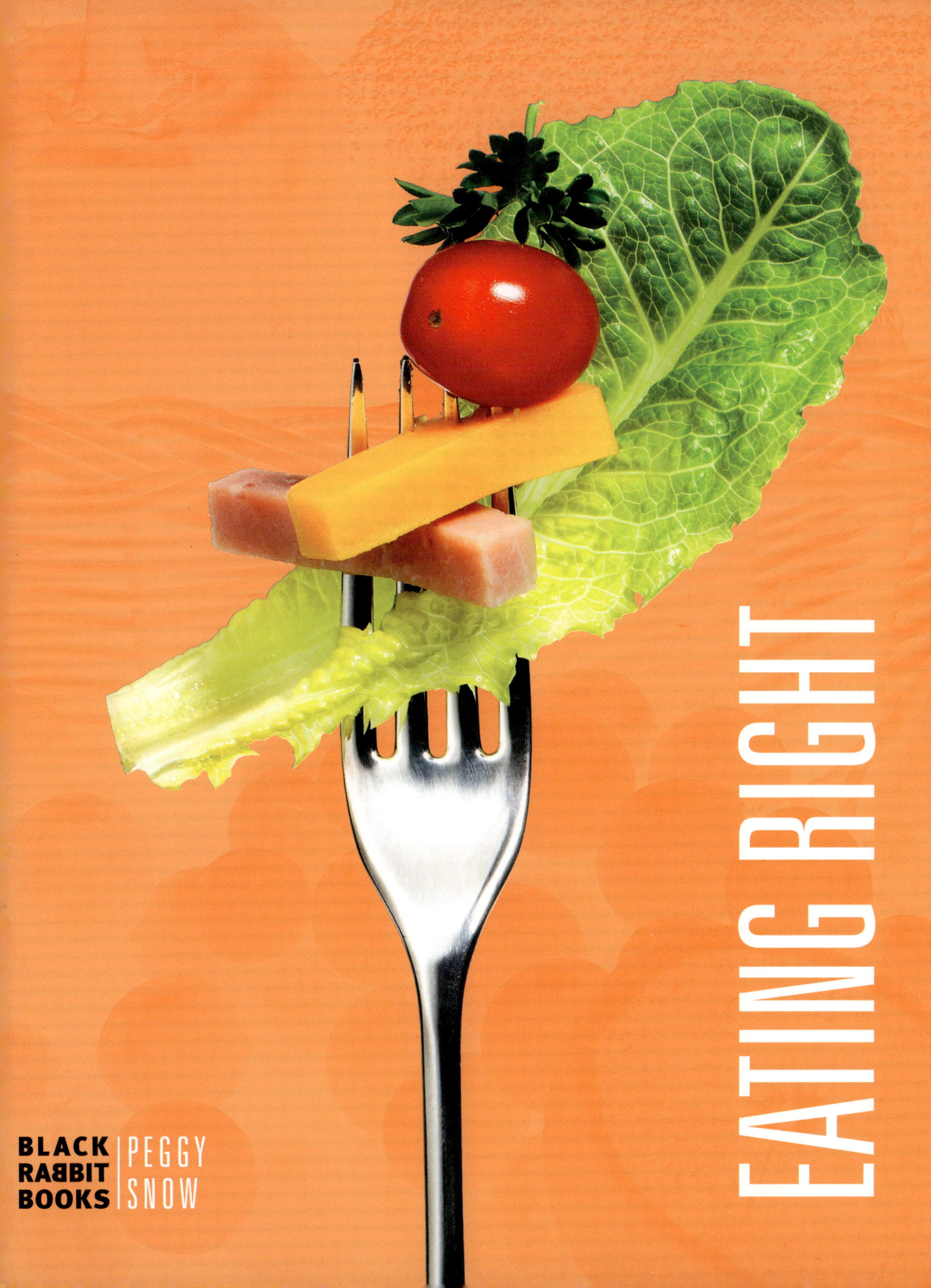
EATING RIGHT
BLACK RABBIT BOOKS
PEGGY SNOW

TABLE OF CONTENTS

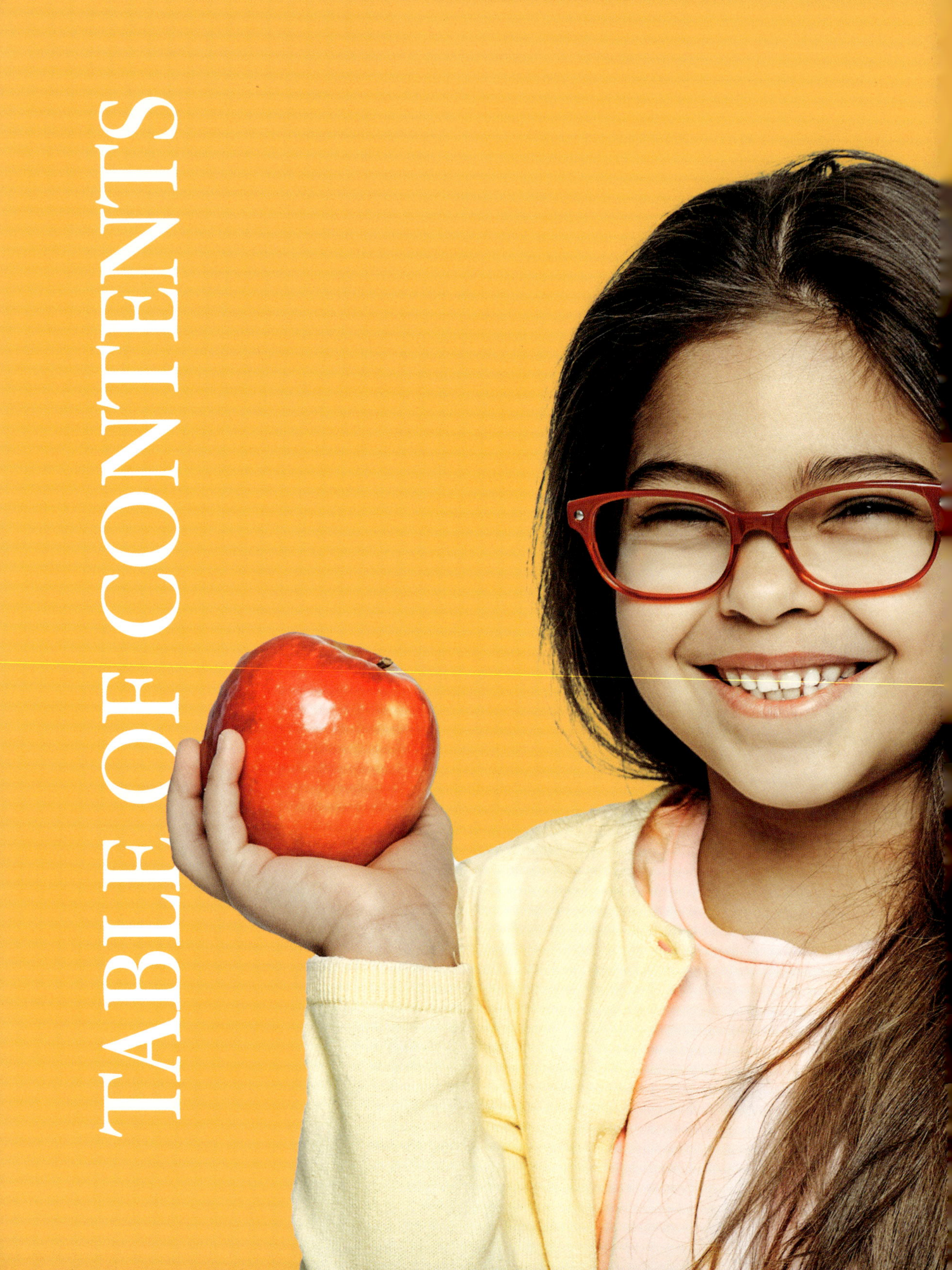

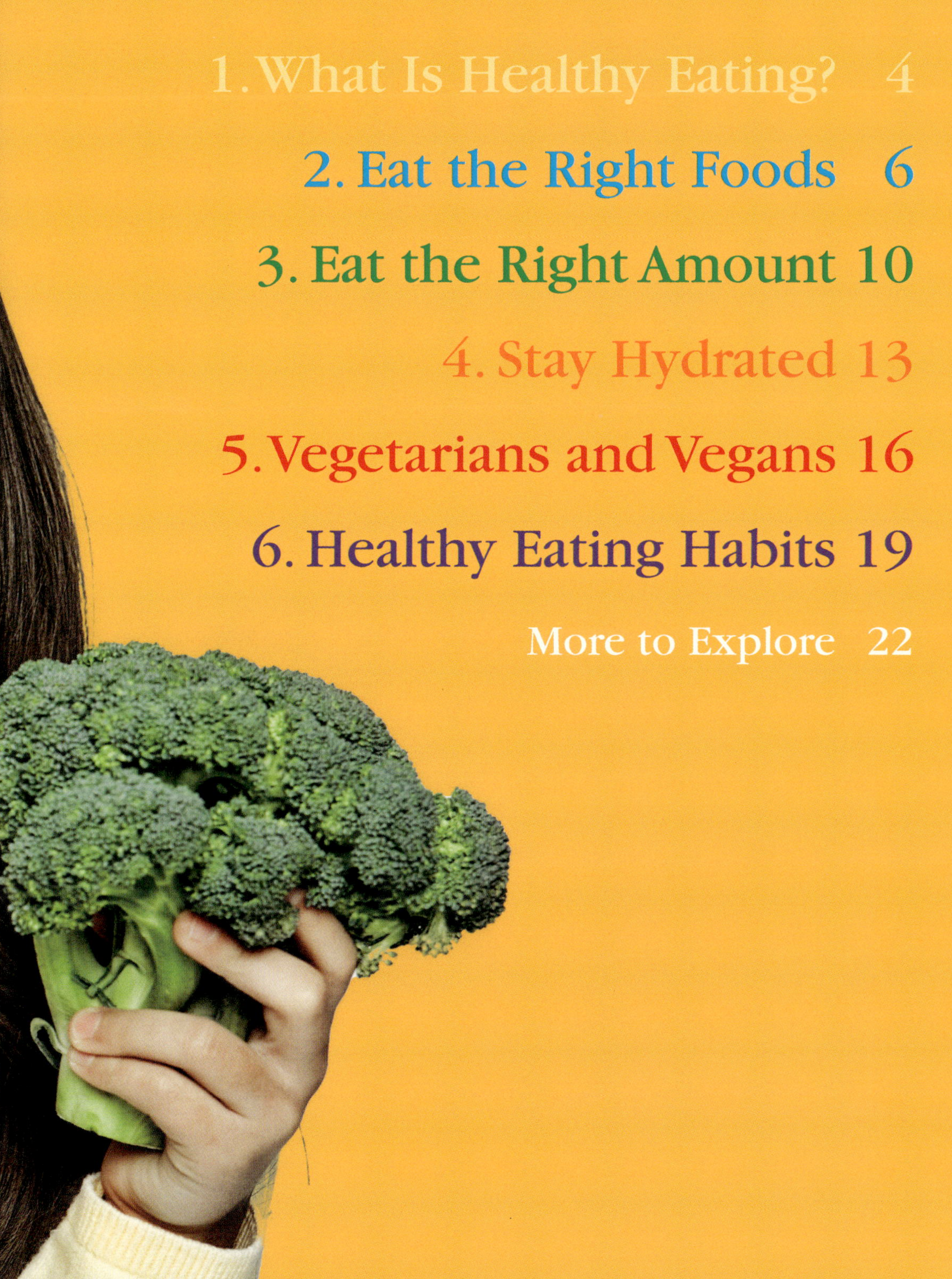

1

What Is Healthy Eating?

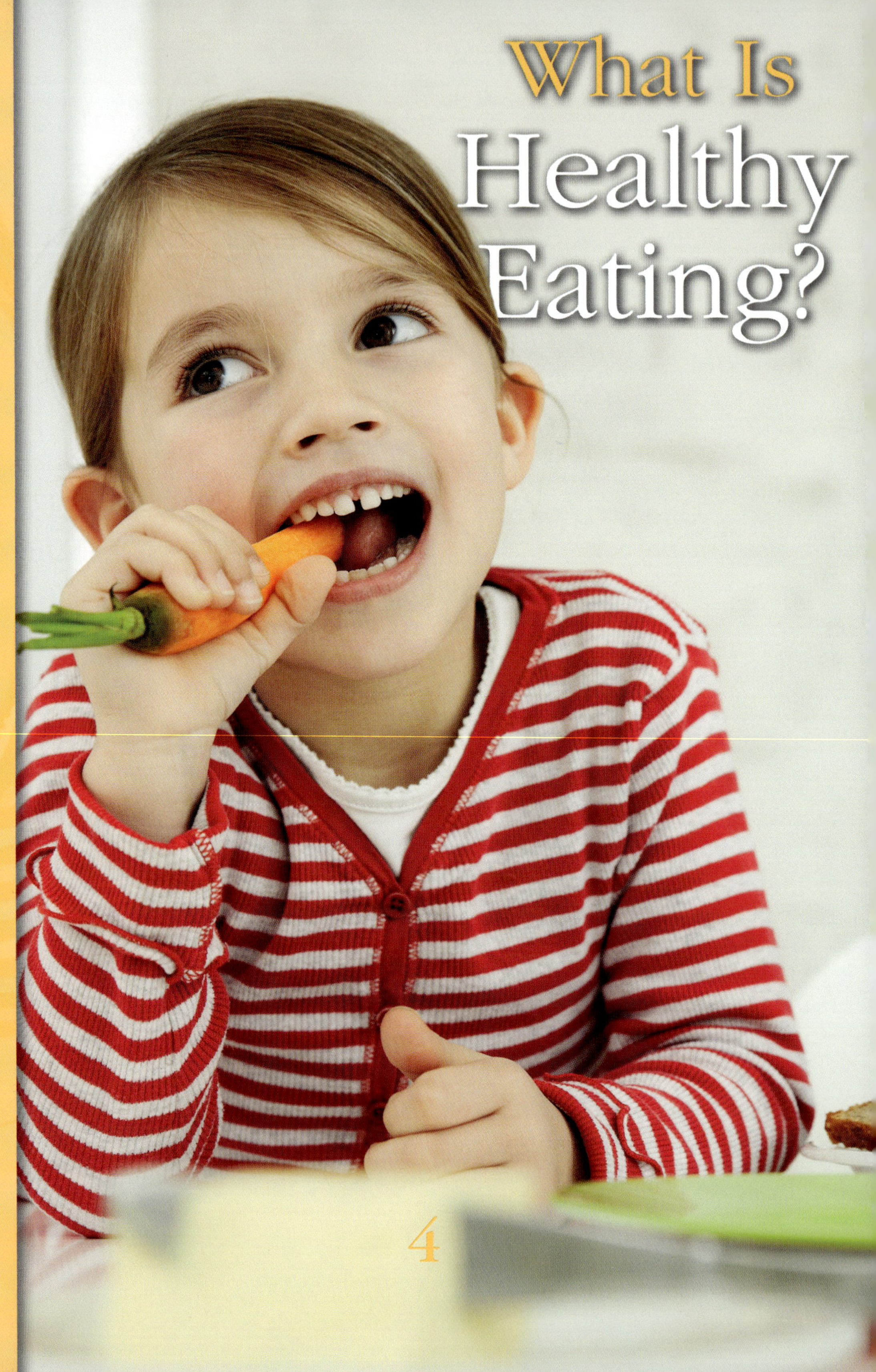

Healthy eating means eating foods that are good for you. Your body needs protein to build muscles. Protein is found in meat, cheese, and beans. Fish, avocados, and eggs give you healthy fat. Whole grains like oatmeal have important nutrients. So do vegetables and fruits.

Healthy foods also have vitamins and minerals. They help protect you from getting sick. It's OK to eat a sugary treat once in a while. But it should not be the only thing you eat.

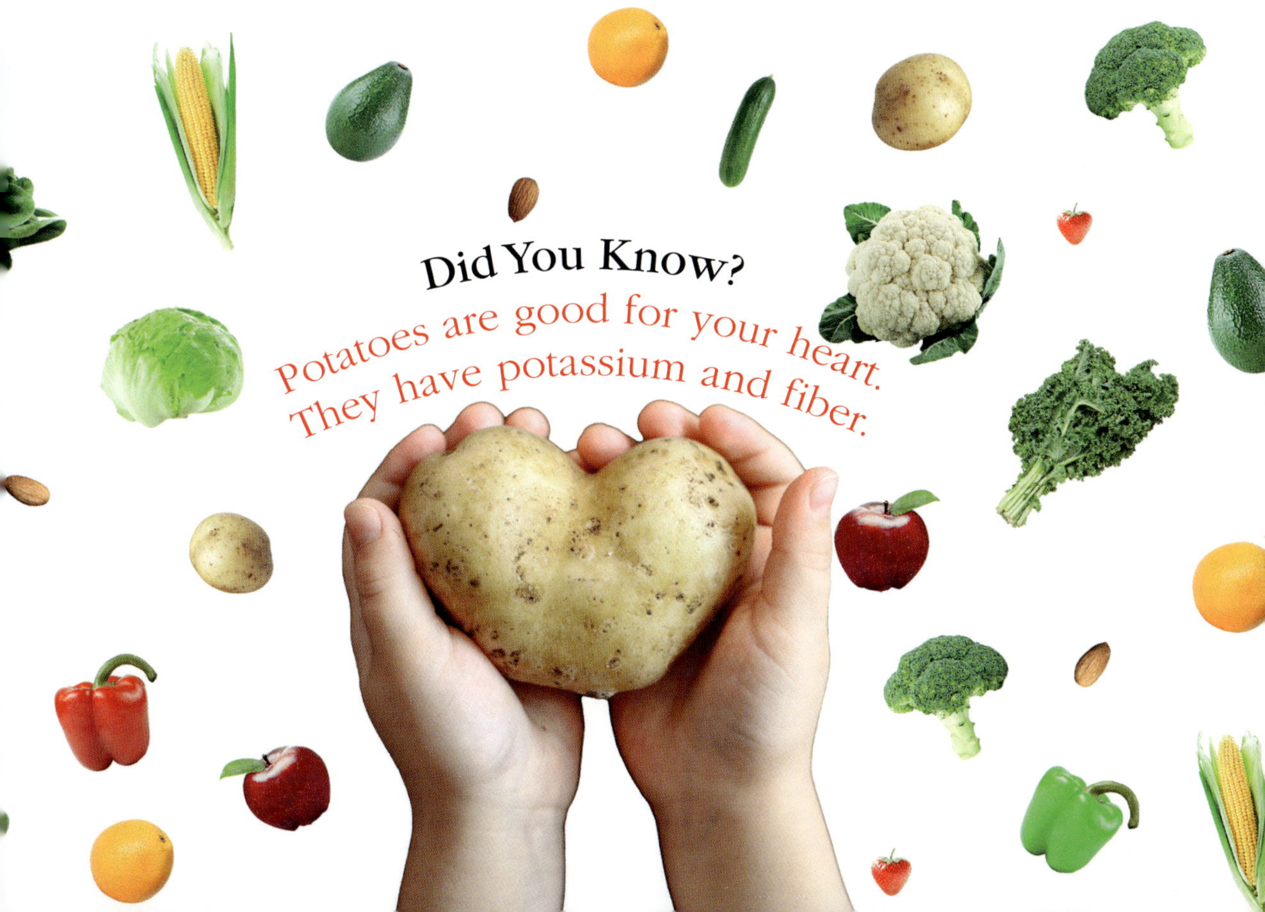

Did You Know?

Potatoes are good for your heart. They have potassium and fiber.

2 Eat the Right Foods

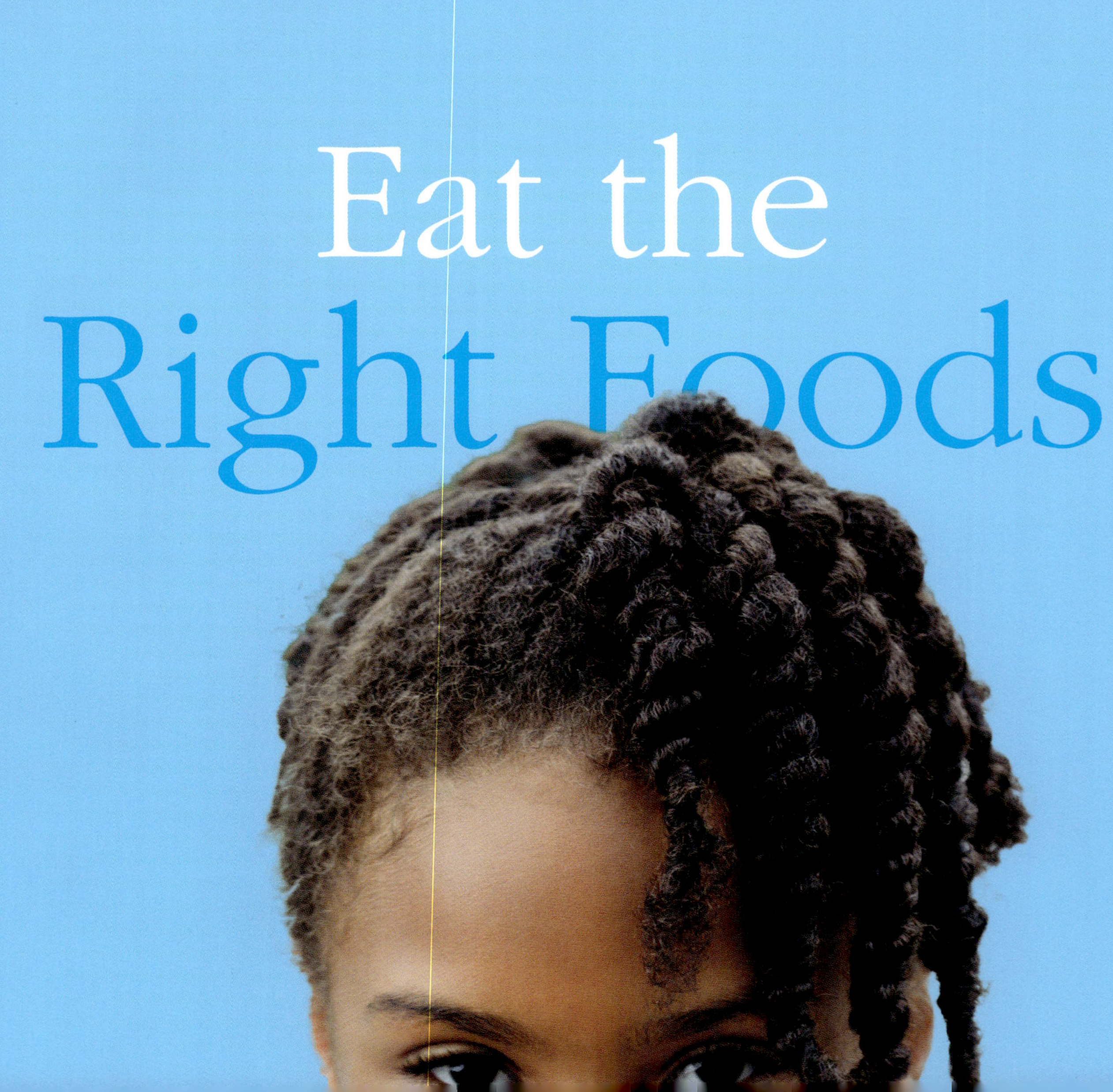

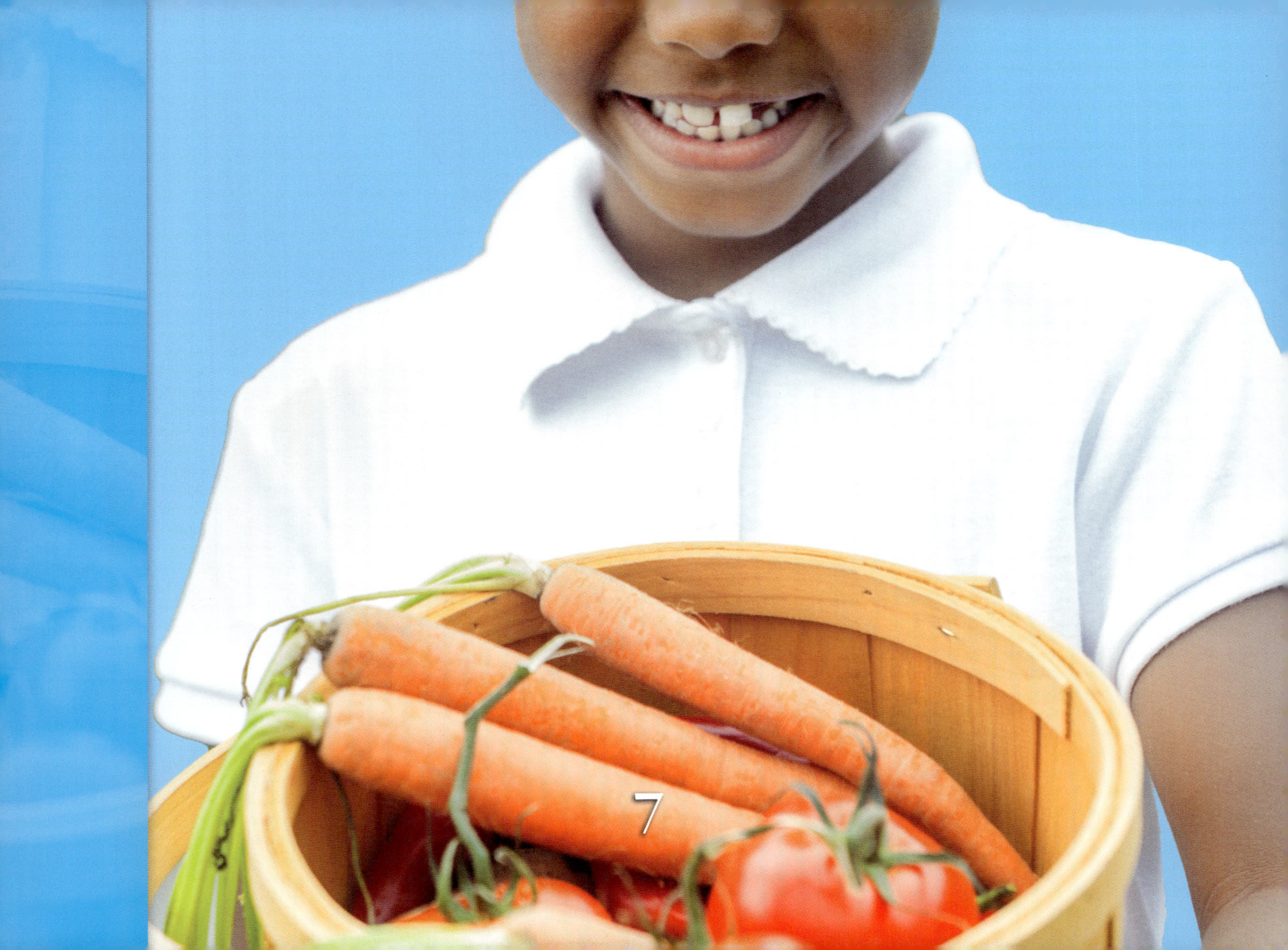

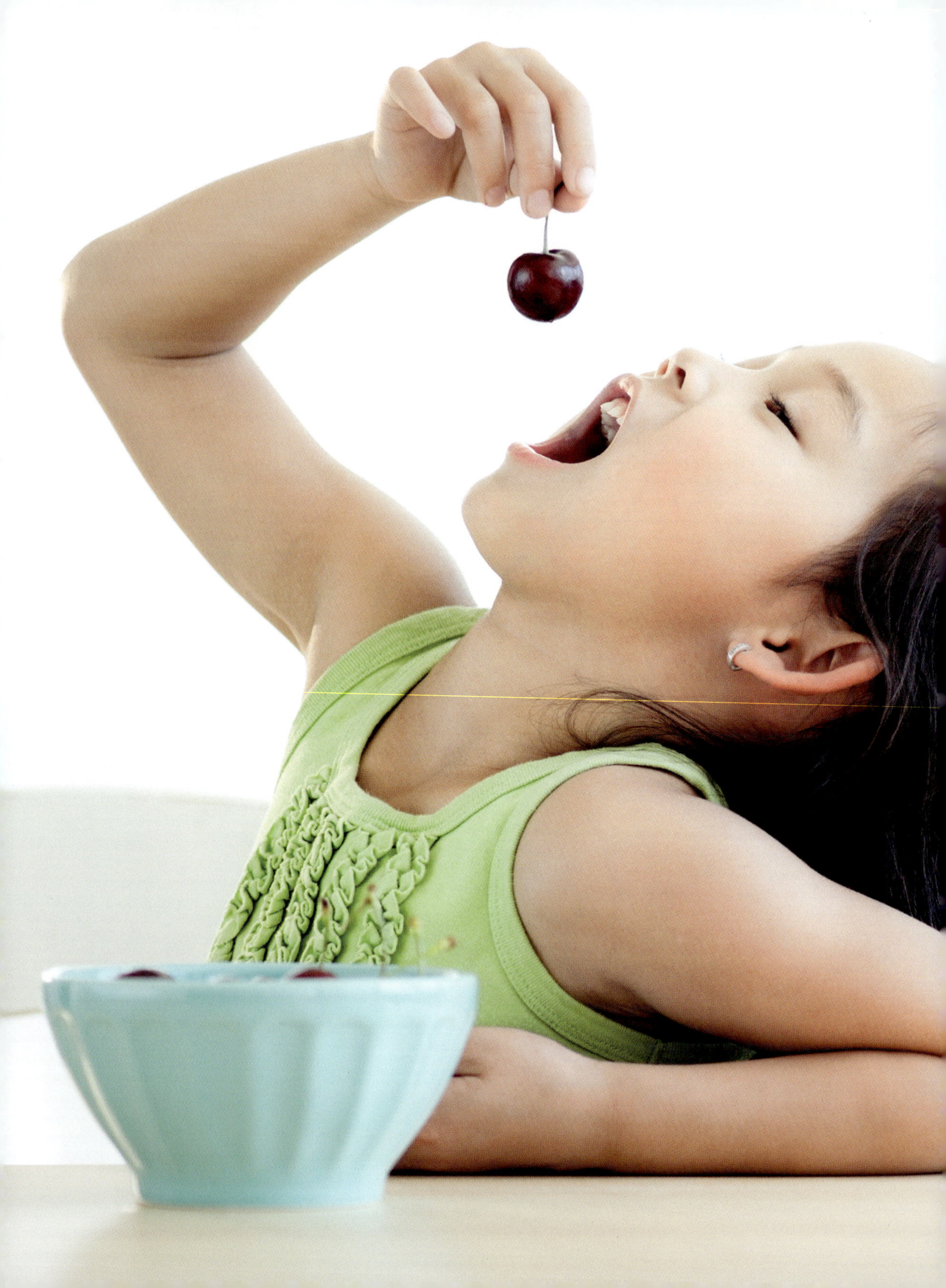

What you put in your stomach affects how you feel. Foods and drinks high in fat or sugar can make you feel tired. Foods rich in vitamins and minerals help you feel good.

Healthy eating gives you energy and improves your mood. Eggs, beans, and yogurt provide energy. Broccoli and blueberries are good for your heart. Walnuts and oranges are good for your brain.

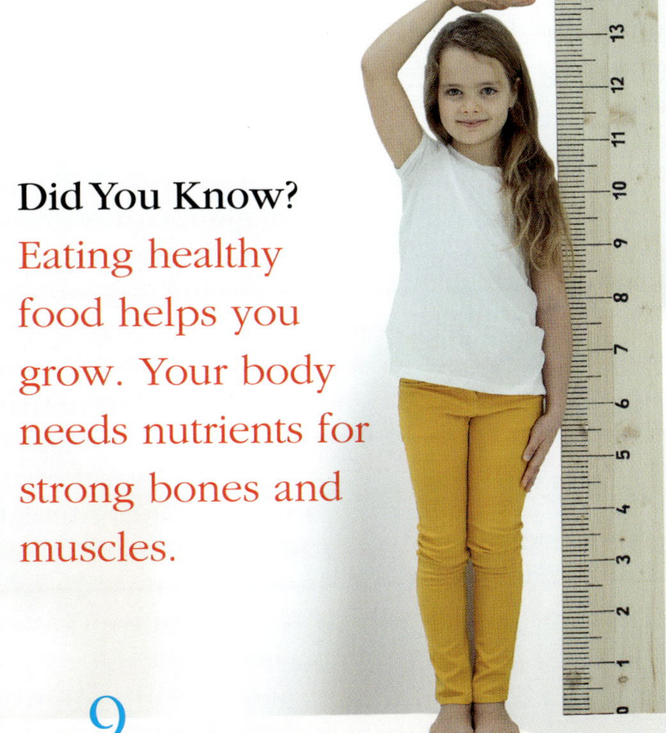

Did You Know?
Eating healthy food helps you grow. Your body needs nutrients for strong bones and muscles.

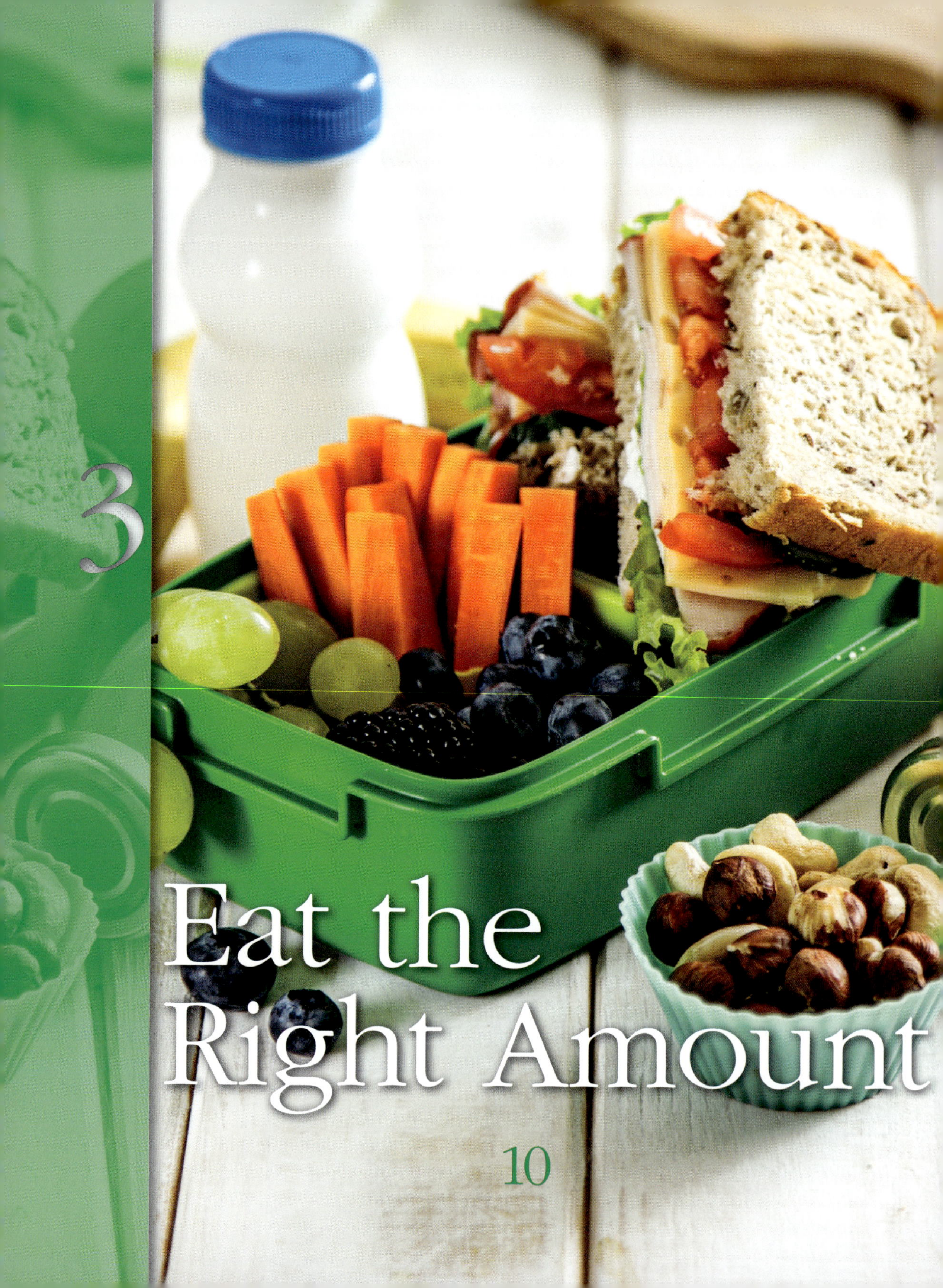

3

Eat the Right Amount

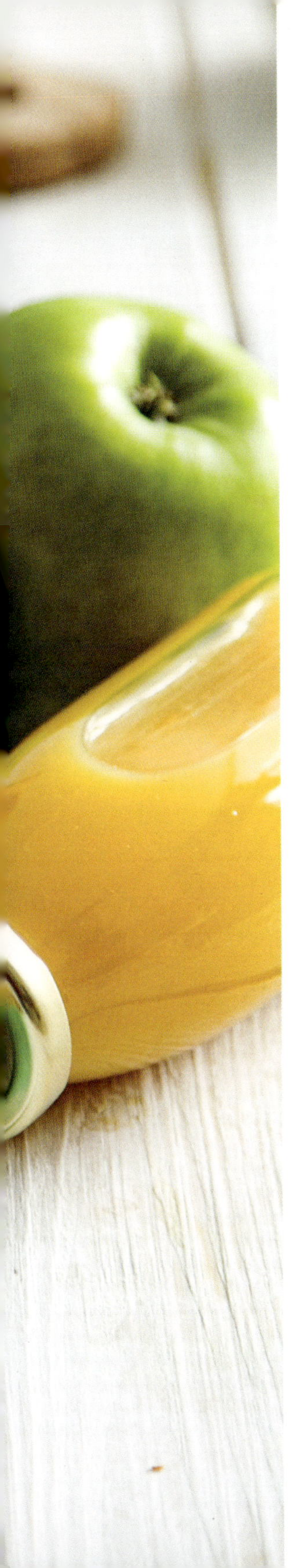

Kids need three meals a day, plus one or two snacks. The more active you are, the more calories you need.

If your stomach is telling you it's hungry, then your body needs nutrients. Skipping meals lowers your energy. It gets harder to think and focus.

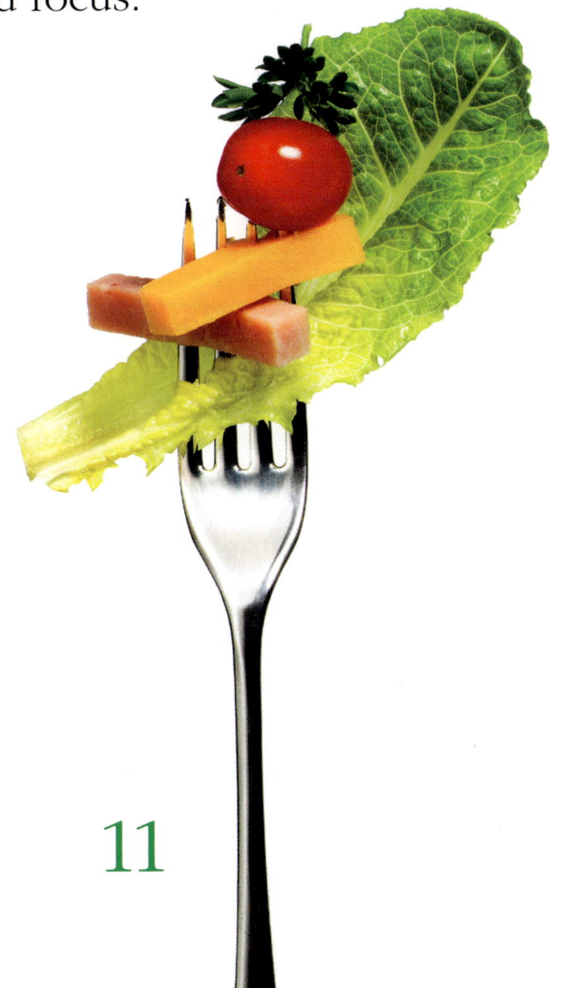

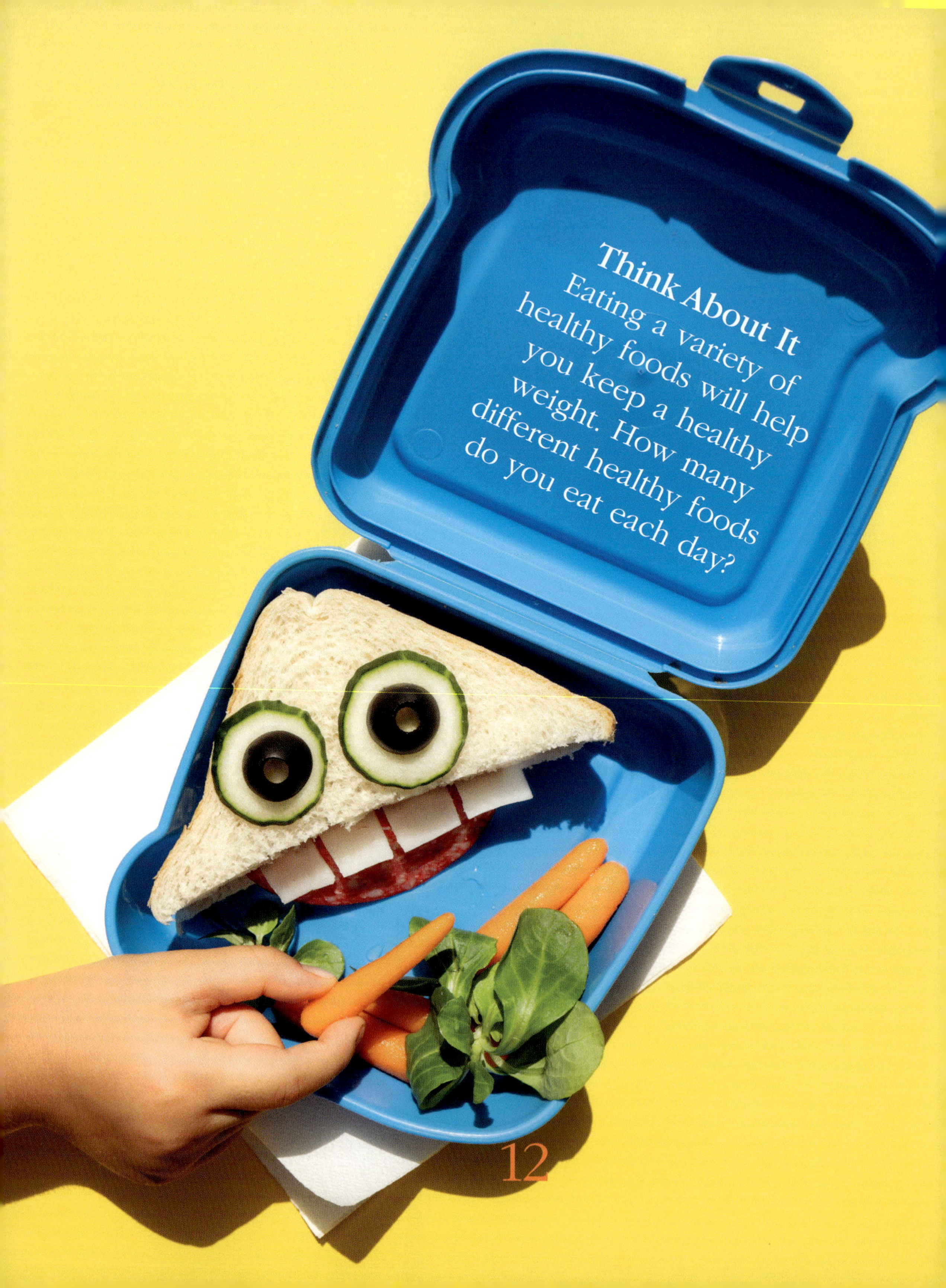
Think About It
Eating a variety of healthy foods will help you keep a healthy weight. How many different healthy foods do you eat each day?

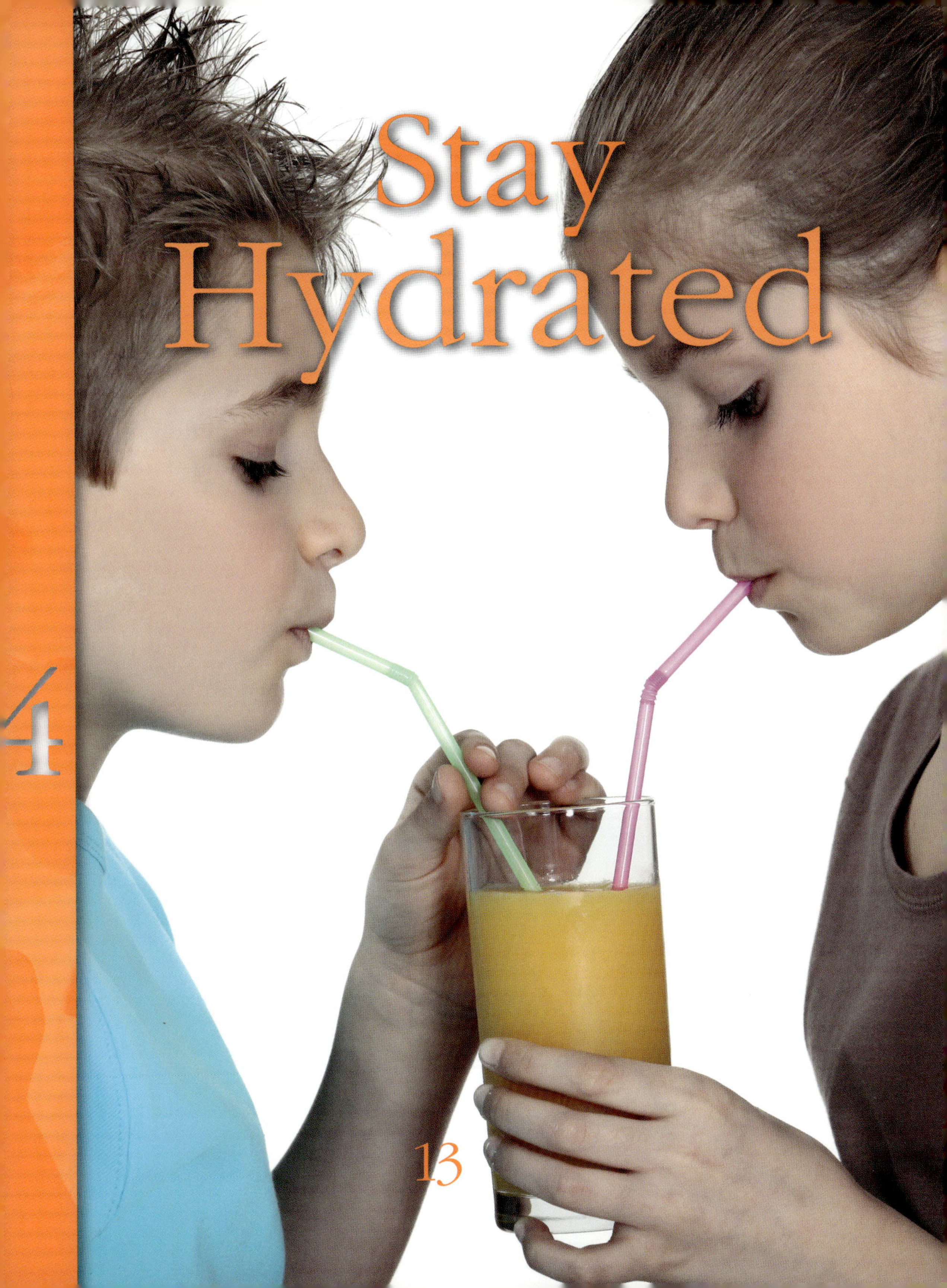

4

Stay Hydrated

Your body is 60 percent water. For everything to work, you need to stay **hydrated**.

You get water from foods like fruits and vegetables. Drinking liquids like water and milk is also important.

Kids need about a half gallon (2 liters) of liquid each day. That is about 8 cups. If you are playing, you need more. You lose water in sweat.

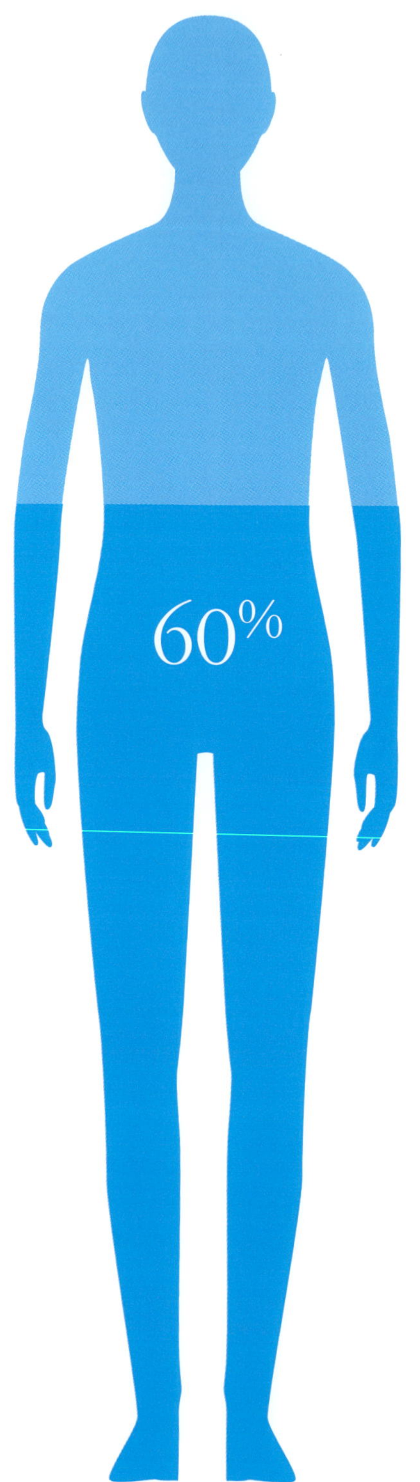

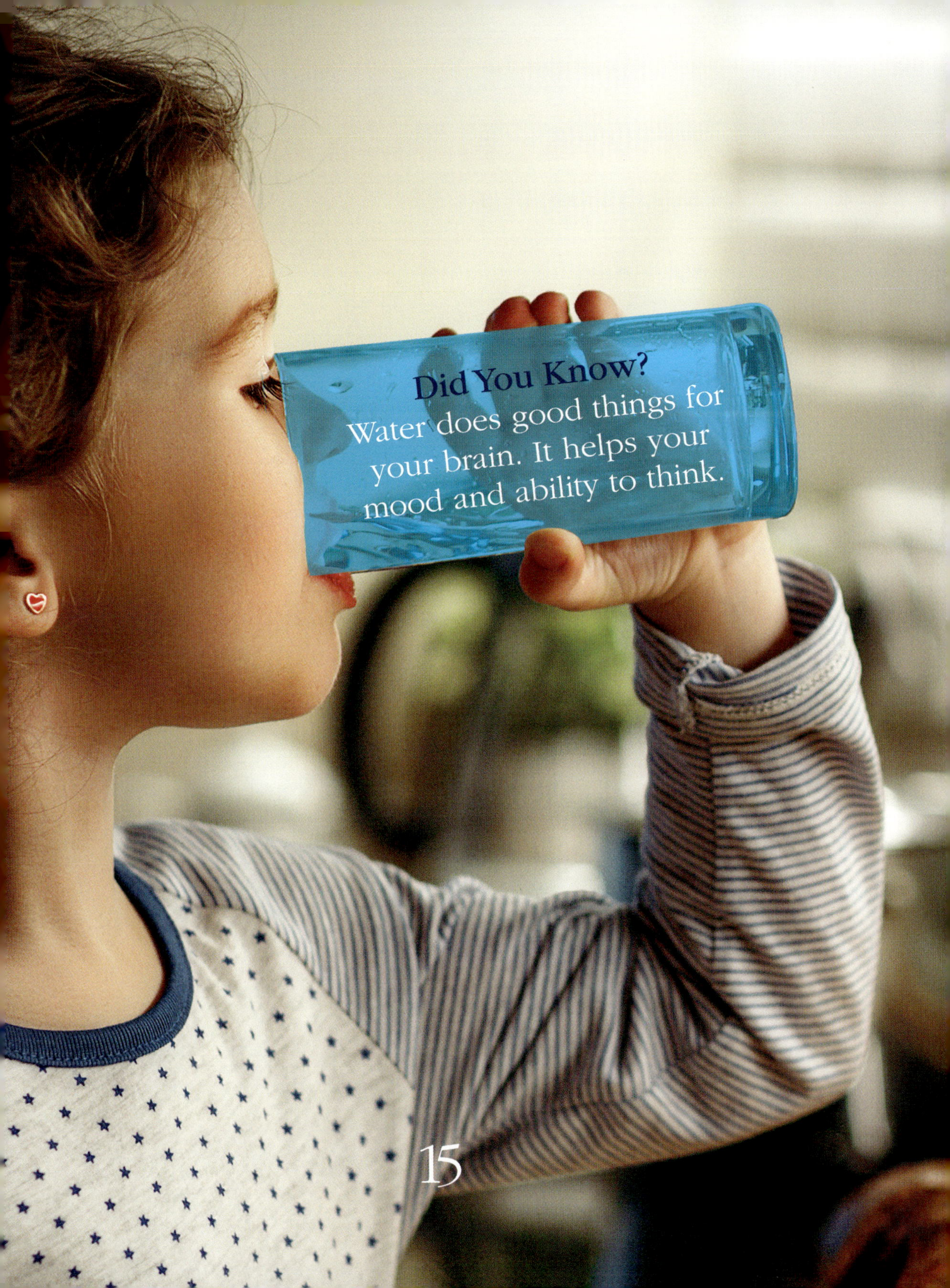
Did You Know?
Water does good things for your brain. It helps your mood and ability to think.

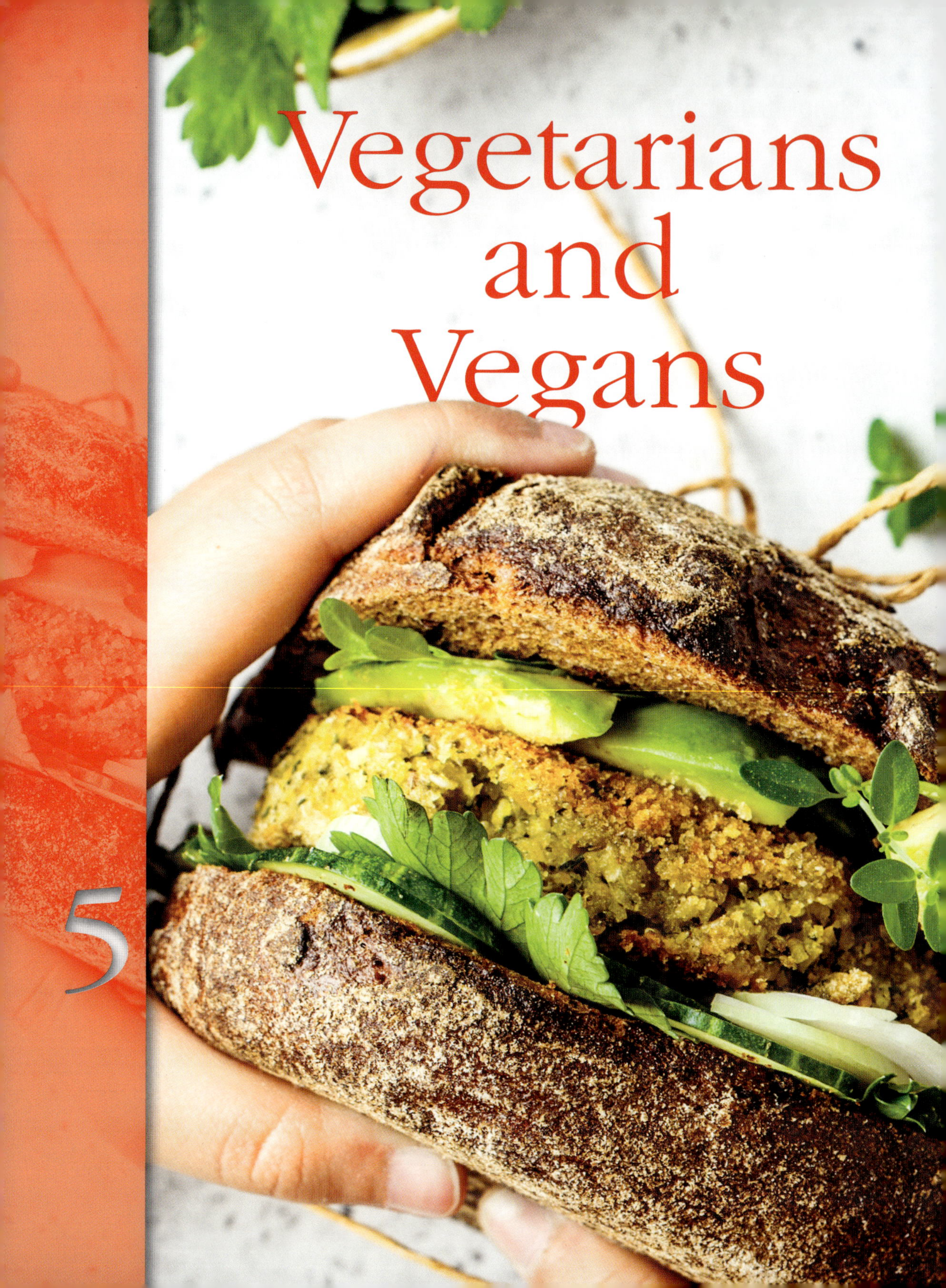

5

Vegetarians and Vegans

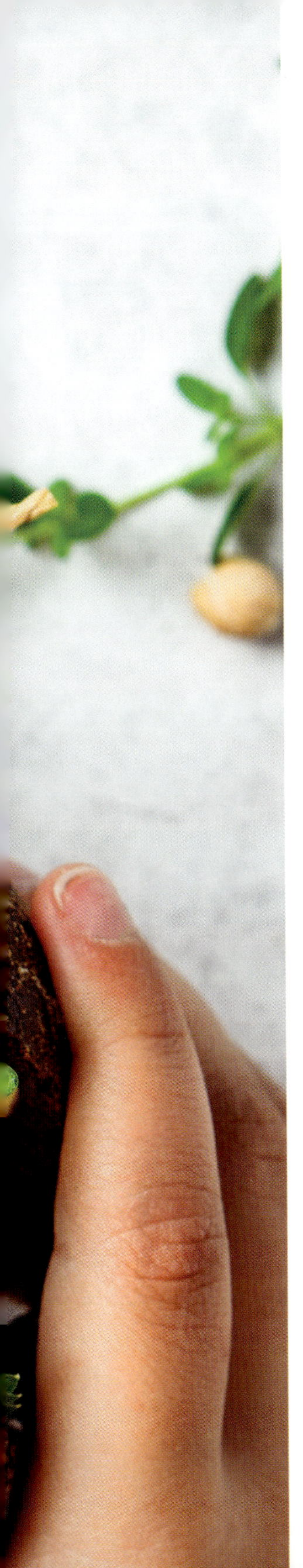

Some people don't eat meat or animal products. They might decide to do this for health reasons. Sometimes it's for religious reasons. Or they do it to save animals or the environment.

Vegetarians don't eat meat. They eat vegetables, fruits, grains, nuts, and legumes. They might eat eggs and dairy products.

Vegans avoid any products from animals. They eat only plant foods. They don't even eat honey because it comes from bees.

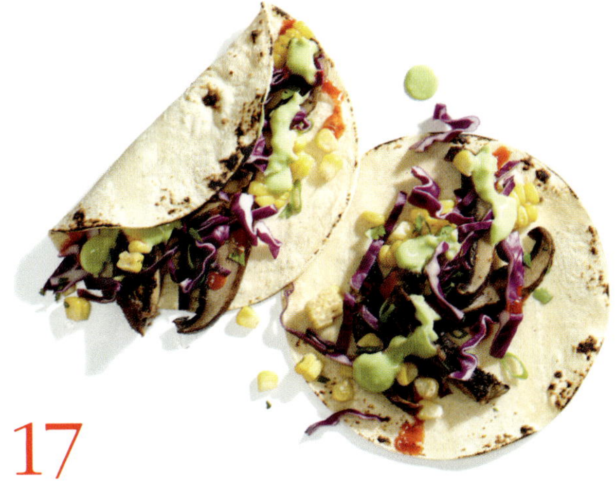

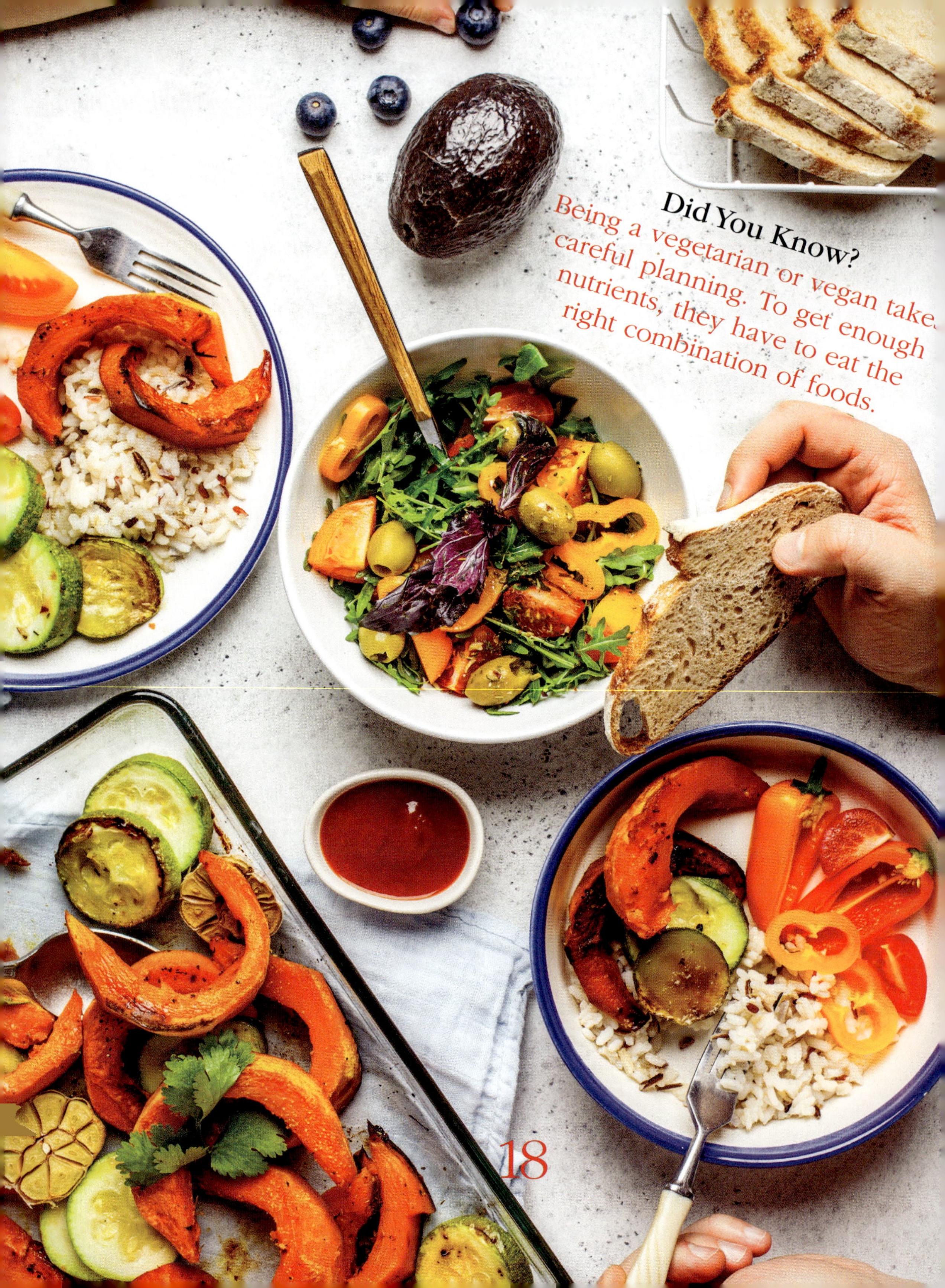

Did You Know?

Being a vegetarian or vegan takes careful planning. To get enough nutrients, they have to eat the right combination of foods.

Healthy Eating Habits

6

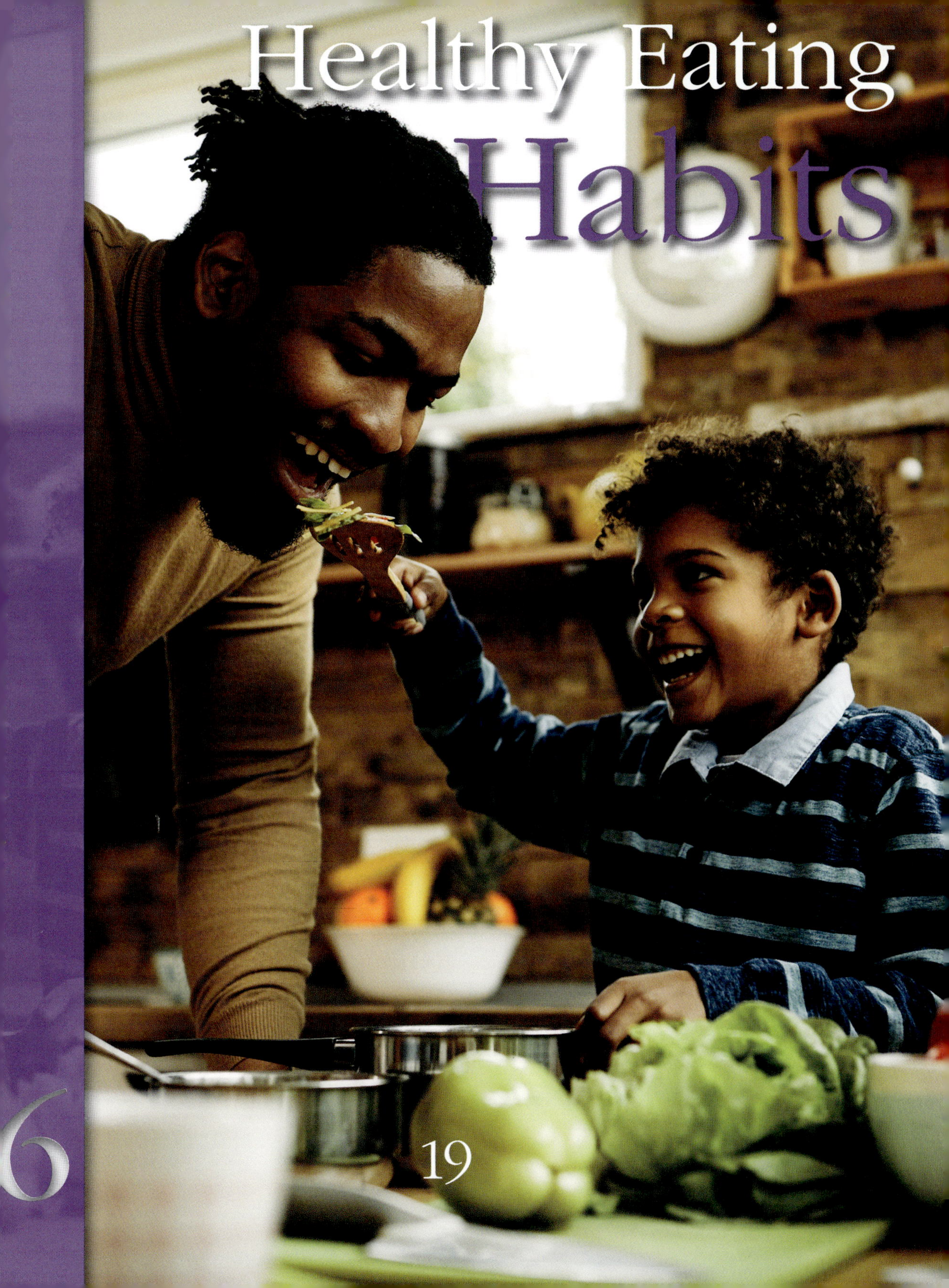

It's easier to eat healthy when you form healthy eating habits. Snack on fruits and veggies instead of junk food. Be willing to try something, even if it looks odd. You may find out you like it!

Ask a parent or caregiver to buy your favorite healthy foods. Try bananas, carrots, cottage cheese, and nuts. Then when you're hungry, the right foods will be in reach.

Help your family plan a meal. You can learn how to chop or fry a food. Cooking can be fun and healthy!

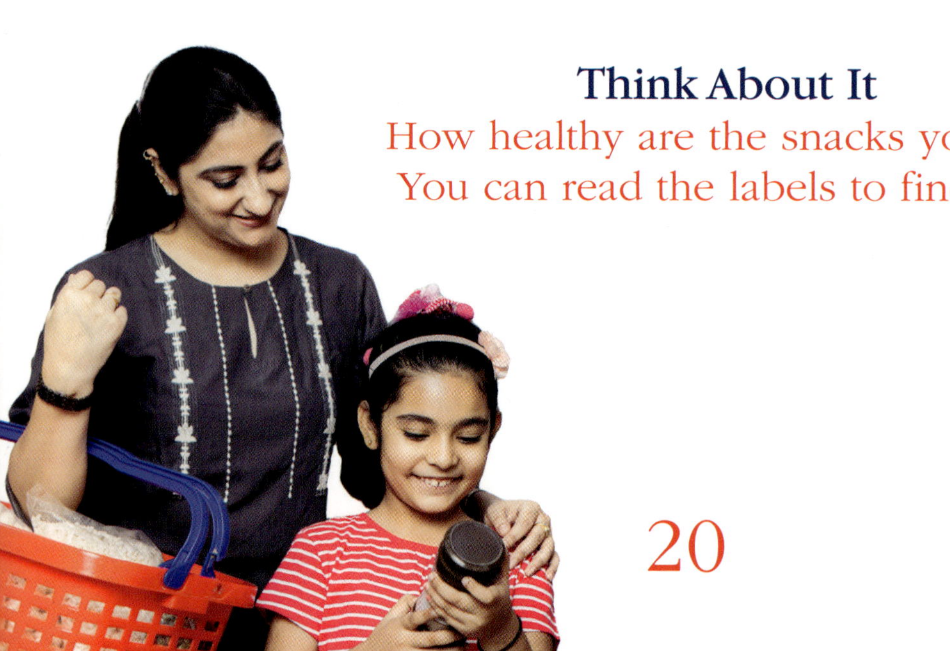

Think About It

How healthy are the snacks you eat? You can read the labels to find out.

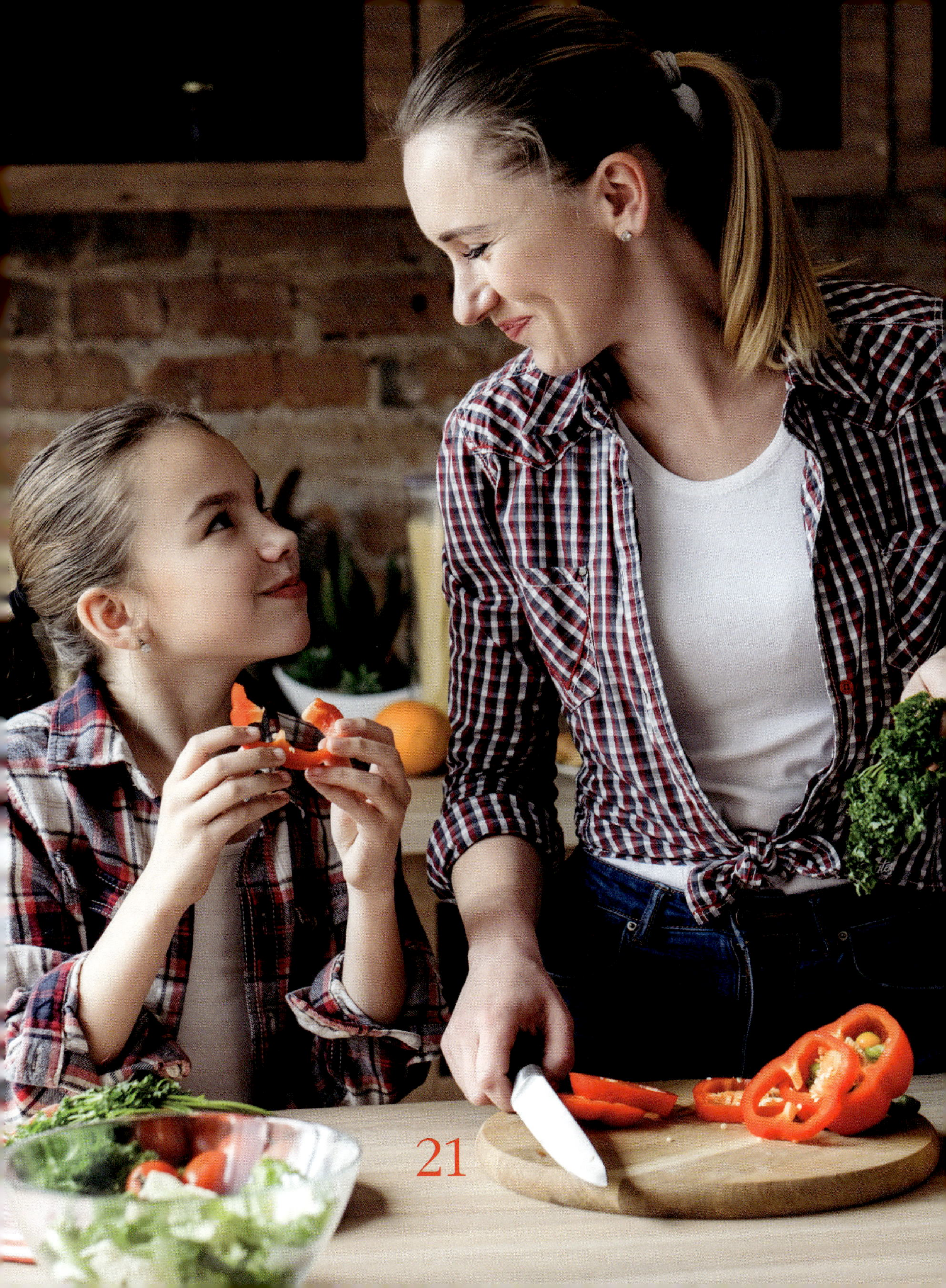

MORE TO EXPLORE

FANTASTIC FACTS

Experts say that children should eat 1–2 servings of fruit and 1–4 servings of vegetables each day.

Eating right can help you live longer.

Cucumbers are 96 percent water. They are a great snack on a hot day!

Five percent of Americans are vegetarians.

A healthy breakfast helps your brain work and gives you energy for the day.

Peanut butter, fruit smoothies, and low-fat cheese are healthy snacks that give you energy.

MORE TO EXPLORE

COOL COMPARISONS

6 unhealthy vs. healthy snacks.

UNHEALTHY	HEALTHY
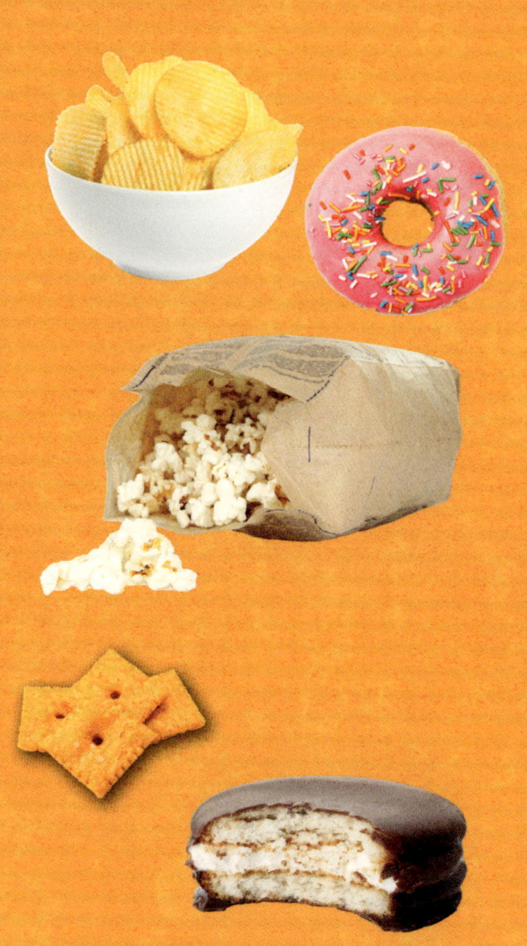	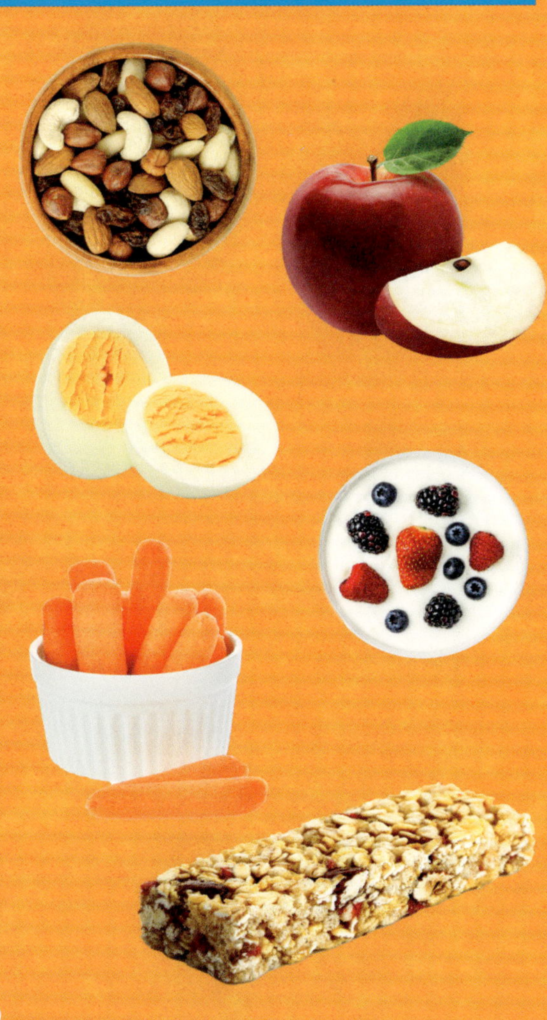

MORE TO EXPLORE

RESOURCES

Glossary

calorie (KAHL-or-eez) A unit of energy that food will give your body.

fiber (FY-buhr) Plant material that cannot be digested.

habit (HAB-it) Something you do on a regular basis.

hydrate (HAHY-dreyt) To supply with water.

legume (leg-YOOM) A vegetable whose seeds are in a pod.

mineral (MINH-er-uhl) A substance found in the ground.

nutrient (NOO-tree-uhnt) A substance in food that is needed to be healthy.

vitamin (VYE-tuh-min) A nutrient found naturally in foods that is needed in smal amounts.

Read More

Bullis, Amber. *Mindfulness and Food.* Minneapolis: Jump!, Inc., 2020.

Chang, Kirsten. *Eating Healthy.* Minneapolis: Bellwether Media, 2022.

Index

TOP RANK is published by Black Rabbit Books, P.O. Box 227, Mankato, MN, 56002.

• Top Rank is an imprint of Black Rabbit Books. • Edited by Alissa Thielges • Designed by Danny Nanos • Photographs © Dreamstime: Phovoir, 13; Getty: Brian Hagiwara, cover, 11, Drazen Zigic, 19, golubovy, 21, JGI/Jamie Grill, 8–9, Ksenia Shestakova, 5, Maren Caruso, 17, oleksii arseniuk, 14, peakSTOCK, 2–3, Realpictures, 20, SDI Productions, 6–7, vaaseenaa, 16, 18, Westend61, 12, 4; Shutterstock: Artem Kutsenko, 23 (apple), Creativa Images, 5, Deenida, 23 (carrots), Evgeny Atamanenko, 15, Kayo, 23 (yogurt), monticello, cover, Moving Moment, 23 (strawberry), Nataliia Pyzhova, 23 (donut), New Africa, 23 (chips, choco pie), Nina Buday, 9, oksana2010, 23 (popcorn), Oleksandra Naumenko, 10–11, Peter Hermes Furian, 23 (nuts), Tiger Images, 23 (cheese crackers), vipman, 23 (egg) • Printed in the United States of America

Library of Congress Cataloging-in-Publication Data: Names: Snow, Peggy, author. | Title: Eating right / by Peggy Snow. | Description: Mankato, MN: Black Rabbit Books, 2025. | Series: Top rank. Healthy and happy | Ages 8–11 | Grades 4–6 | Identifiers: LCCN 2023058222 | ISBN 9781632357960 (library binding) | ISBN 9781645820741 (ebook) | Subjects: LCSH: Nutrition—Juvenile literature. | Health—Juvenile literature. | Classification: LCC RA784 .S5995 2025 | DDC 613.2—dc23/eng/20240110 | LC record available at https://lccn.loc.gov/2023058222